# Essential Oils

## Lists – Oils – Blends – Recipes

This Notebook belongs:

_______________________

# Lists

# My Oils

| Name | Used for | Date opened | Kid safe |
| --- | --- | --- | --- |
|  |  |  |  |
|  |  |  |  |
|  |  |  |  |
|  |  |  |  |
|  |  |  |  |
|  |  |  |  |
|  |  |  |  |
|  |  |  |  |
|  |  |  |  |
|  |  |  |  |
|  |  |  |  |
|  |  |  |  |
|  |  |  |  |
|  |  |  |  |
|  |  |  |  |
|  |  |  |  |
|  |  |  |  |

| Name | Used for | Date opened | Kid safe |
| --- | --- | --- | --- |
|  |  |  |  |
|  |  |  |  |
|  |  |  |  |
|  |  |  |  |
|  |  |  |  |
|  |  |  |  |
|  |  |  |  |
|  |  |  |  |
|  |  |  |  |
|  |  |  |  |
|  |  |  |  |
|  |  |  |  |
|  |  |  |  |
|  |  |  |  |
|  |  |  |  |
|  |  |  |  |
|  |  |  |  |
|  |  |  |  |
| Name | Used for | Date opened | Kid safe |
|  |  |  |  |
|  |  |  |  |
|  |  |  |  |
|  |  |  |  |

| Name | Used for | Date opened | Kid safe |
| --- | --- | --- | --- |
|  |  |  |  |
|  |  |  |  |
|  |  |  |  |
|  |  |  |  |
|  |  |  |  |
|  |  |  |  |
|  |  |  |  |
|  |  |  |  |
|  |  |  |  |
|  |  |  |  |
|  |  |  |  |
|  |  |  |  |
|  |  |  |  |
|  |  |  |  |
|  |  |  |  |
|  |  |  |  |
|  |  |  |  |
|  |  |  |  |
|  |  |  |  |
|  |  |  |  |
|  |  |  |  |
|  |  |  |  |

# My Wish List

| Name | Used for | Date order | Get it |
| --- | --- | --- | --- |
|  |  |  |  |
|  |  |  |  |
|  |  |  |  |
|  |  |  |  |
|  |  |  |  |
|  |  |  |  |
|  |  |  |  |
|  |  |  |  |
|  |  |  |  |
|  |  |  |  |
|  |  |  |  |
|  |  |  |  |
|  |  |  |  |
|  |  |  |  |
|  |  |  |  |
|  |  |  |  |
|  |  |  |  |

| Name | Used for | Date order | Get it |
| --- | --- | --- | --- |
|  |  |  |  |
|  |  |  |  |
|  |  |  |  |
|  |  |  |  |
|  |  |  |  |
|  |  |  |  |
|  |  |  |  |
|  |  |  |  |
|  |  |  |  |
|  |  |  |  |
|  |  |  |  |
|  |  |  |  |
|  |  |  |  |
|  |  |  |  |
|  |  |  |  |
|  |  |  |  |
|  |  |  |  |
|  |  |  |  |
|  |  |  |  |
|  |  |  |  |
|  |  |  |  |
|  |  |  |  |
|  |  |  |  |
|  |  |  |  |

| Name | Used for | Date order | Get it |
|------|----------|------------|--------|
|      |          |            |        |
|      |          |            |        |
|      |          |            |        |
|      |          |            |        |
|      |          |            |        |
|      |          |            |        |
|      |          |            |        |
|      |          |            |        |
|      |          |            |        |
|      |          |            |        |
|      |          |            |        |
|      |          |            |        |
|      |          |            |        |
|      |          |            |        |
|      |          |            |        |
|      |          |            |        |
|      |          |            |        |
|      |          |            |        |

# My Favorite Oils

| Name | Used for | Date opened | Kid safe |
| --- | --- | --- | --- |
|  |  |  |  |
|  |  |  |  |
|  |  |  |  |
|  |  |  |  |
|  |  |  |  |
|  |  |  |  |
|  |  |  |  |
|  |  |  |  |
|  |  |  |  |
|  |  |  |  |
|  |  |  |  |
|  |  |  |  |
|  |  |  |  |
|  |  |  |  |
|  |  |  |  |
|  |  |  |  |
|  |  |  |  |
|  |  |  |  |

| Name | Used for | Date opened | Kid safe |
| --- | --- | --- | --- |
|  |  |  |  |
|  |  |  |  |
|  |  |  |  |
|  |  |  |  |
|  |  |  |  |
|  |  |  |  |
|  |  |  |  |
|  |  |  |  |
|  |  |  |  |
|  |  |  |  |
|  |  |  |  |
|  |  |  |  |
|  |  |  |  |
|  |  |  |  |
|  |  |  |  |
|  |  |  |  |
|  |  |  |  |
|  |  |  |  |
|  |  |  |  |
|  |  |  |  |
|  |  |  |  |
|  |  |  |  |
|  |  |  |  |
|  |  |  |  |

| Name | Used for | Date opened | Kid safe |
| --- | --- | --- | --- |
|  |  |  |  |
|  |  |  |  |
|  |  |  |  |
|  |  |  |  |
|  |  |  |  |
|  |  |  |  |
|  |  |  |  |
|  |  |  |  |
|  |  |  |  |
|  |  |  |  |
|  |  |  |  |
|  |  |  |  |
|  |  |  |  |
|  |  |  |  |
|  |  |  |  |
|  |  |  |  |
|  |  |  |  |
| Name | Used for | Date opened | Kid safe |
|  |  |  |  |
|  |  |  |  |
|  |  |  |  |

# My oils

Oil

☐ Topical          ☐ Aromatical          ☐ Internal

Tips/Uses:

Oil

☐ Topical          ☐ Aromatical          ☐ Internal

Tips/Uses:

Oil

☐ Topical          ☐ Aromatical          ☐ Internal

Tips/Uses:

Oil

☐ Topical          ☐ Aromatical          ☐ Internal

Tips/Uses:

Oil

☐ Topical          ☐ Aromatical          ☐ Internal

Tips/Uses:

Oil

☐ Topical          ☐ Aromatical          ☐ Internal

Tips/Uses:

Oil

☐ Topical          ☐ Aromatical          ☐ Internal

Tips/Uses:

Oil

☐ Topical          ☐ Aromatical          ☐ Internal

Tips/Uses:

Oil

☐ Topical          ☐ Aromatical          ☐ Internal

Tips/Uses:

Oil

☐ Topical  ☐ Aromatical  ☐ Internal

Tips/Uses:

Oil

☐ Topical     ☐ Aromatical     ☐ Internal

Tips/Uses:

Oil

☐ Topical          ☐ Aromatical          ☐ Internal

Tips/Uses:

Oil

☐ Topical　　　☐ Aromatical　　　☐ Internal

Tips/Uses:

Oil

☐ Topical          ☐ Aromatical          ☐ Internal

Tips/Uses:

Oil

☐ Topical          ☐ Aromatical          ☐ Internal

Tips/Uses:

Oil

☐ Topical ☐ Aromatical ☐ Internal

Tips/Uses:

Oil

☐ Topical            ☐ Aromatical            ☐ Internal

Tips/Uses:

Oil

☐ Topical      ☐ Aromatical      ☐ Internal

Tips/Uses:

Oil

☐ Topical        ☐ Aromatical        ☐ Internal

Tips/Uses:

Oil

☐ Topical          ☐ Aromatical          ☐ Internal

Tips/Uses:

Oil

☐ Topical          ☐ Aromatical          ☐ Internal

Tips/Uses:

Oil

☐ Topical     ☐ Aromatical     ☐ Internal

Tips/Uses:

Oil

☐ Topical   ☐ Aromatical   ☐ Internal

Tips/Uses:

Oil

☐ Topical          ☐ Aromatical          ☐ Internal

Tips/Uses:

Oil

☐ Topical    ☐ Aromatical    ☐ Internal

Tips/Uses:

Oil

☐ Topical          ☐ Aromatical          ☐ Internal

Tips/Uses:

Oil

☐ Topical          ☐ Aromatical          ☐ Internal

Tips/Uses:

Oil

☐ Topical          ☐ Aromatical          ☐ Internal

Tips/Uses:

Oil

☐ Topical          ☐ Aromatical          ☐ Internal

Tips/Uses:

Oil

☐ Topical       ☐ Aromatical       ☐ Internal

Tips/Uses:

Oil

☐ Topical          ☐ Aromatical          ☐ Internal

Tips/Uses:

Oil

☐ Topical          ☐ Aromatical          ☐ Internal

Tips/Uses:

Oil

☐ Topical          ☐ Aromatical          ☐ Internal

Tips/Uses:

Oil

☐ Topical          ☐ Aromatical          ☐ Internal

Tips/Uses:

Oil

☐ Topical          ☐ Aromatical          ☐ Internal

Tips/Uses:

Oil

☐ Topical     ☐ Aromatical     ☐ Internal

Tips/Uses:

Oil

☐ Topical          ☐ Aromatical          ☐ Internal

Tips/Uses:

Oil

☐ Topical          ☐ Aromatical          ☐ Internal

Tips/Uses:

Oil

☐ Topical          ☐ Aromatical          ☐ Internal

Tips/Uses:

Oil

☐ Topical          ☐ Aromatical          ☐ Internal

Tips/Uses:

Oil

☐ Topical      ☐ Aromatical      ☐ Internal

Tips/Uses:

Oil

☐ Topical  ☐ Aromatical  ☐ Internal

Tips/Uses:

Oil

☐ Topical          ☐ Aromatical          ☐ Internal

Tips/Uses:

Oil

☐ Topical          ☐ Aromatical          ☐ Internal

Tips/Uses:

Oil

☐ Topical          ☐ Aromatical          ☐ Internal

Tips/Uses:

Oil

☐ Topical          ☐ Aromatical          ☐ Internal

Tips/Uses:

Oil

☐ Topical          ☐ Aromatical          ☐ Internal

Tips/Uses:

Oil

☐ Topical          ☐ Aromatical          ☐ Internal

Tips/Uses:

Oil

☐ Topical          ☐ Aromatical          ☐ Internal

Tips/Uses:

Oil

☐ Topical          ☐ Aromatical          ☐ Internal

Tips/Uses:

Oil

☐ Topical          ☐ Aromatical          ☐ Internal

Tips/Uses:

Oil

☐ Topical          ☐ Aromatical          ☐ Internal

Tips/Uses:

Oil

☐ Topical          ☐ Aromatical          ☐ Internal

Tips/Uses:

Oil

☐ Topical          ☐ Aromatical          ☐ Internal

Tips/Uses:

Oil

☐ Topical          ☐ Aromatical          ☐ Internal

Tips/Uses:

Oil

☐ Topical          ☐ Aromatical          ☐ Internal

Tips/Uses:

Oil

☐ Topical          ☐ Aromatical          ☐ Internal

Tips/Uses:

Oil

☐ Topical          ☐ Aromatical          ☐ Internal

Tips/Uses:

Oil

☐ Topical          ☐ Aromatical          ☐ Internal

Tips/Uses:

Oil

☐ Topical          ☐ Aromatical          ☐ Internal

Tips/Uses:

Oil

☐ Topical          ☐ Aromatical          ☐ Internal

Tips/Uses:

Oil

☐ Topical          ☐ Aromatical          ☐ Internal

Tips/Uses:

Oil

☐ Topical          ☐ Aromatical          ☐ Internal

Tips/Uses:

Oil

☐ Topical ☐ Aromatical ☐ Internal

Tips/Uses:

Oil

☐ Topical          ☐ Aromatical          ☐ Internal

Tips/Uses:

Oil

☐ Topical ☐ Aromatical ☐ Internal

Tips/Uses:

Oil

☐ Topical  ☐ Aromatical  ☐ Internal

Tips/Uses:

Oil

☐ Topical      ☐ Aromatical      ☐ Internal

Tips/Uses:

Oil

☐ Topical          ☐ Aromatical          ☐ Internal

Tips/Uses:

Oil

☐ Topical  ☐ Aromatical  ☐ Internal

Tips/Uses:

Oil

☐ Topical ☐ Aromatical ☐ Internal

Tips/Uses:

Oil

☐ Topical          ☐ Aromatical          ☐ Internal

Tips/Uses:

# Blends

Blend:

☐ Topical ☐ Aromatical ☐ Internal

Tips/Uses:

Blend:

☐ Topical          ☐ Aromatical          ☐ Internal

Tips/Uses:

Blend:

☐ Topical    ☐ Aromatical    ☐ Internal

Tips/Uses:

Blend:

☐ Topical          ☐ Aromatical          ☐ Internal

Tips/Uses:

Blend:

☐ Topical  ☐ Aromatical  ☐ Internal

Tips/Uses:

Blend:

☐ Topical          ☐ Aromatical          ☐ Internal

Tips/Uses:

Blend:

☐ Topical          ☐ Aromatical          ☐ Internal

Tips/Uses:

Blend:

☐ Topical          ☐ Aromatical          ☐ Internal

Tips/Uses:

Blend:

☐ Topical    ☐ Aromatical    ☐ Internal

Tips/Uses:

Blend:

☐ Topical    ☐ Aromatical    ☐ Internal

Tips/Uses:

Blend:

☐ Topical          ☐ Aromatical          ☐ Internal

Tips/Uses:

Blend:

☐ Topical          ☐ Aromatical          ☐ Internal

Tips/Uses:

Blend:

☐ Topical  ☐ Aromatical  ☐ Internal

Tips/Uses:

Blend:

☐ Topical          ☐ Aromatical          ☐ Internal

Tips/Uses:

Blend:

☐ Topical    ☐ Aromatical    ☐ Internal

Tips/Uses:

Blend:

☐ Topical          ☐ Aromatical          ☐ Internal

Tips/Uses:

Blend:

☐ Topical          ☐ Aromatical          ☐ Internal

Tips/Uses:

Blend:

☐ Topical          ☐ Aromatical          ☐ Internal

Tips/Uses:

Blend:

☐ Topical          ☐ Aromatical          ☐ Internal

Tips/Uses:

Blend:

☐ Topical          ☐ Aromatical          ☐ Internal

Tips/Uses:

Blend:

☐ Topical  ☐ Aromatical  ☐ Internal

Tips/Uses:

Blend:

☐ Topical          ☐ Aromatical          ☐ Internal

Tips/Uses:

Blend:

☐ Topical  ☐ Aromatical  ☐ Internal

Tips/Uses:

Blend:

☐ Topical          ☐ Aromatical          ☐ Internal

Tips/Uses:

Blend:

☐ Topical    ☐ Aromatical    ☐ Internal

Tips/Uses:

Blend:

☐ Topical          ☐ Aromatical          ☐ Internal

Tips/Uses:

Blend:

☐ Topical     ☐ Aromatical     ☐ Internal

Tips/Uses:

Blend:

☐ Topical          ☐ Aromatical          ☐ Internal

Tips/Uses:

Blend:

☐ Topical      ☐ Aromatical      ☐ Internal

Tips/Uses:

Blend:

☐ Topical          ☐ Aromatical          ☐ Internal

Tips/Uses:

Blend:

☐ Topical          ☐ Aromatical          ☐ Internal

Tips/Uses:

Blend:

☐ Topical          ☐ Aromatical          ☐ Internal

Tips/Uses:

Blend:

☐ Topical          ☐ Aromatical          ☐ Internal

Tips/Uses:

Blend:

☐ Topical          ☐ Aromatical          ☐ Internal

Tips/Uses:

Blend:

☐ Topical          ☐ Aromatical          ☐ Internal

Tips/Uses:

Blend:

☐ Topical          ☐ Aromatical          ☐ Internal

Tips/Uses:

Blend:

☐ Topical          ☐ Aromatical          ☐ Internal

Tips/Uses:

Blend:

☐ Topical          ☐ Aromatical          ☐ Internal

Tips/Uses:

Blend:

☐ Topical  ☐ Aromatical  ☐ Internal

Tips/Uses:

Blend:

☐ Topical　　　☐ Aromatical　　　☐ Internal

Tips/Uses:

# Diy Recipes

Diy Recipes:

☐ Body  ☐ Home  ☐ Children  ☐ ________

You need:

Tips/Uses:

Diy Recipes:

☐ Body   ☐ Home   ☐ Children   ☐ _________

You need:

Tips/Uses:

Diy Recipes:

☐ Body    ☐ Home    ☐ Children    ☐ ________

You need:

Tips/Uses:

Diy Recipes:

☐ Body   ☐ Home   ☐ Children   ☐ __________

You need:

Tips/Uses:

Diy Recipes:

☐ Body  ☐ Home  ☐ Children  ☐ ________

You need:

Tips/Uses:

Diy Recipes:

☐ Body  ☐ Home  ☐ Children  ☐ __________

You need:

Tips/Uses:

Diy Recipes:

☐ Body  ☐ Home  ☐ Children  ☐ ________

You need:

Tips/Uses:

Diy Recipes:

☐ Body  ☐ Home  ☐ Children  ☐ _________

You need:

Tips/Uses:

Diy Recipes:

☐ Body  ☐ Home  ☐ Children  ☐ _________

You need:

Tips/Uses:

Diy Recipes:

☐ Body   ☐ Home   ☐ Children   ☐ _________

You need:

Tips/Uses:

Diy Recipes:

☐ Body   ☐ Home   ☐ Children   ☐ _________

You need:

Tips/Uses:

Diy Recipes:

☐ Body    ☐ Home    ☐ Children    ☐ __________

You need:

Tips/Uses:

Diy Recipes:

☐ Body    ☐ Home    ☐ Children    ☐ _________

You need:

Tips/Uses:

Diy Recipes:

☐ Body   ☐ Home   ☐ Children   ☐ __________

You need:

Tips/Uses:

Diy Recipes:

☐ Body  ☐ Home  ☐ Children  ☐ ________

You need:

Tips/Uses:

Diy Recipes:

☐ Body   ☐ Home   ☐ Children   ☐ _________

You need:

Tips/Uses:

Diy Recipes:

☐ Body    ☐ Home    ☐ Children    ☐ _________

You need:

Tips/Uses:

Diy Recipes:

☐ Body   ☐ Home   ☐ Children   ☐ _________

You need:

Tips/Uses:

Diy Recipes:

☐ Body  ☐ Home  ☐ Children  ☐ _________

You need:

Tips/Uses:

Diy Recipes:

☐ Body    ☐ Home    ☐ Children    ☐ ________

You need:

Tips/Uses:

Diy Recipes:

☐ Body   ☐ Home   ☐ Children   ☐ _________

You need:

Tips/Uses:

Diy Recipes:

☐ Body  ☐ Home  ☐ Children  ☐ _________

You need:

Tips/Uses:

Diy Recipes:

☐ Body    ☐ Home    ☐ Children    ☐ __________

You need:

Tips/Uses:

Diy Recipes:

☐ Body    ☐ Home    ☐ Children    ☐ __________

You need:

Tips/Uses:

Diy Recipes:

☐ Body   ☐ Home   ☐ Children   ☐ _________

You need:

Tips/Uses:

Diy Recipes:

☐ Body   ☐ Home   ☐ Children   ☐ _________

You need:

Tips/Uses:

DIY Recipes:

☐ Body   ☐ Home   ☐ Children   ☐ _________

You need:

Tips/Uses:

Diy Recipes:

☐ Body  ☐ Home  ☐ Children  ☐ _________

You need:

Tips/Uses:

Diy Recipes:

☐ Body   ☐ Home   ☐ Children   ☐ _________

You need:

Tips/Uses:

Diy Recipes:

☐ Body  ☐ Home  ☐ Children  ☐ _________

You need:

Tips/Uses:

Diy Recipes:

☐ Body  ☐ Home  ☐ Children  ☐ ________

You need:

Tips/Uses:

Diy Recipes:

☐ Body　　☐ Home　　☐ Children　　☐ _________

You need:


Tips/Uses:

Diy Recipes:

☐ Body　　☐ Home　　☐ Children　　☐ ________

You need:

Tips/Uses:

DIY Recipes:

☐ Body    ☐ Home    ☐ Children    ☐ __________

You need:

Tips/Uses:

Diy Recipes:

☐ Body    ☐ Home    ☐ Children    ☐ _________

You need:

Tips/Uses:

Diy Recipes:

☐ Body   ☐ Home   ☐ Children   ☐ __________

You need:

Tips/Uses:

Diy Recipes:

☐ Body    ☐ Home    ☐ Children    ☐ ________

You need:

Tips/Uses:

Diy Recipes:

☐ Body    ☐ Home    ☐ Children    ☐ _________

You need:

Tips/Uses:

Diy Recipes:

☐ Body   ☐ Home   ☐ Children   ☐ ________

You need:

Tips/Uses:

Diy Recipes:

☐ Body  ☐ Home  ☐ Children  ☐ ___________

You need:

Tips/Uses:

Diy Recipes:

☐ Body  ☐ Home  ☐ Children  ☐ _________

You need:

Tips/Uses:

# Notes